Of course
I have cancer.
Who doesn't?

PHYLLIS JOHNSTON

DEDICATION

To my incomparable males and female triumvirate

CONTENTS

ACKNOWLEDGMENTS

Cancer is not something I navigate alone. From the diagnosis through all the treatments there were outstanding oncologists, caring radiology techs, the absolute greatest chemo nurses, the welcoming Tammy and the indescribably fantastic Liz.

From the onset of this life-changing event, my incomparable support triumvirate—Pamela, Mary Ellen and Joanne—remain steadfast, caring and funny. And then there are my males. Jake, the Wheaton Terrier, who continues to sleep beside me, ready to make me laugh or give me a kiss. Ben—aka the perfect husband (yes, really)—gives me joy, comfort, Reiki and damn good home cooked meals.

Special thanks to Sasha for nudging me to write this and providing ridiculously honest comments on the text, and to Steve and George for being such caring friends to Ben.

I will forever be grateful for having these remarkable people in my life and hope I can pay forward at least some of the inestimable gifts they continue to give to me.

1 GETTING A GRIP

Yes, I have cancer. So do nearly fourteen million other people. And in 2013 another 1.7 million will become members of the club they never wanted to join.

Yes, cancer is the second most common cause of death in America. Despite this impressive mortality ranking, cancer is a mere common noun in the hierarchy of diseases. Unlike the initial cap diseases—Alzheimer's, Multiple Sclerosis, Parkinson's, Lou Gehrig's—not even one of the more than one hundred sixty types of cancer merits an upper case "c".

Yes, the current five-year survival rate for all cancers is sixty-eight percent. Good for them. For me, the survival rate is twenty percent. Not so good for me. But does that statistic set me apart from the larger cancer crowd? Hardly, according to the late great Christopher Hitchins. After being diagnosed with esophageal cancer, which has a survival rate of five percent, Hitchins commented he was a "member of a cancer elite" who found himself "looking down on people with lesser cancers".

I keep thinking having the most lethal form of the deadliest type of cancer should merit some special recognition in the Little C Club. Not a chance.

Some five months after I was diagnosed, Michael Douglas announced he had Stage IV throat cancer. He underwent chemo and radiation, and within five months, presto, the tumor was gone. Who can compete with that? His wife, actually, the effervescent actress Catherine Zeta-Jones who took over the headlines with her inability to rejoice in her husband's tumor-free status due to her own Bipolar II Disorder (please note the initial caps).

Now as I write this I read someone has garnered not only a place on the April *New York Times* Bestseller List, but also landed a movie deal for her humorous and heart rending book about living life to its fullest before being consumed by Lou Gehrig's Disease. Don't get me wrong. I have great empathy and respect for this bold and talented woman. But couldn't she have waited until I finished my witty and touching account, or perhaps recorded her manuscript rather than typing most of it on her iPhone using only her right thumb?

The bottom line is simple—having cancer does not make me special or unique. It does make me frequently tired, sometimes sad and always overweight, even now after three years. But the breath grabbing, heart palpitating terror is gone, replaced by an all-out effort to fuggedaboutit. This may sound simplistic and maybe it is, but it sure beats the hell out of waking up each morning wondering if today is the day I will die.

2 MY REIKI MASTER

Ben and I have been together for nearly three decades. By now, I should know everything there is to know about him. Wrong.

At the conclusion of the rapid-fire diagnosis process, we stood in our living room holding on to each other. We had, in just more than a week, lost so very much of our lives. We were devastated, wiped out, barely moving under the oppressive weight of sadness. Then Ben made a simple pronouncement that changed the you're-gonna-die-soon paradigm.

"The doctors will do their best, but I will heal you."

"I'm very happy to hear that, but exactly how are you going to do it?" Despite my best efforts, a smattering of incredulity broke through.

"Reiki. I have been studying Reiki on my own for a number of years and I will complete a course to become a Reiki master in just a few more weeks."

I knew nothing about Reiki, but I know my

husband. If he says he's going to heal me using Reiki, I believe him.

He began almost daily Reiki treatments. I just laid down, fully clothed, on Ben's new massage table, closed my eyes and tried to meditate. (I'm still working on the meditation thing.) Ben placed his hands lightly on my body, moving from head to toe to facilitate the healing response. This is akin to placing your hands where it hurts when you are experiencing pain.

Each treatment gave me back control of my mind and body for a minimum of sixty minutes—some days much longer. The duration of being pain- and stress-free paled in comparison to the sense I was in control of my breathing. I was in control of exhaling at the site of the pain. I was in control of letting the healing move throughout my body. This was—and continues to be—priceless.

ABCs of Reiki

Reiki (pronounced *ray key*) is derived from two Japanese words: *rei*, or universal and *ki*, or life energy. This ancient technique, "rediscovered" by Dr. Mikao Usui in Japan during the early twentieth century, has now spread throughout the world.

Reiki promotes the body's innate healing abilities to reduce pain and stress, boost the immune system and promote overall health. It is also used by people seeking relief from disease-related symptoms and the side effects of conventional medical treatments, such as chemotherapy and radiation.

Reiki complements and enhances the health care provided in hospitals and medical clinics. In fact, Reiki is incorporated into cancer, AIDS, pain management and stress/relaxation treatments offered at more than fifty leading hospitals throughout the country, including Memorial Sloan Kettering Cancer Center and Dana-Farber Cancer Institute.

3 SELECTING THE CIRCLE

When I was diagnosed in late March 2010, I decided to tell as few people as possible and strictly on a need-to-know basis. Besides my husband Ben, I told just eight other people. Three were "my women" who came to help during my treatment, a former neighbor with ties to the oncology community, two people I was working with on specific assignments and two neighbors. I asked each one to promise not to tell anyone because:

- I loathe being sick;
- I detest being pitied;
- I lack the grace to accept sympathy; and
- the cancer stigma is a sure-fire way to end a consultant's career. (I am living proof of that.)

In kinder, gentler moments I explained my sphere of silence is imposed for the good of others. Really, what can they do to improve my health and/or Ben's wellbeing? Why would I want them to shoulder this knowledge? Better to let this one go unrevealed.

Besides, most people don't have a clue as to what to say when confronted with such declarative statements as

"I have small cell lung cancer. I have a twenty percent chance of surviving five years." In my limited experience, most start crying. I know I did.

When I called my sister to ask her to fly out in a few weeks to be with us during what my oncologists termed the most difficult period of the combined chemotherapy and radiation regime, I first had to explain my illness. She sobbed.

"Pamela, I am so flattered by your response, but now I need you to stop crying and focus. There'll be time to cry later." I have yet to see her cry, but I know she does.

The few people I told tended to be tongue-tied. Not knowing the right thing to say often leads to platitudes—I'm so sorry, you look great, I know you can beat this. If this is the best someone can conjure up when cold cocked with the cancer news, I'd suggest giving me a hug and keeping quiet.

It would be very helpful if people could understand that from my perspective, "I'm so very sorry" is what you say when confronted with hopelessness or attending a funeral.

"You look great" is either a lie or a remark from a blind person. I aged five years during the first year. You can race matchbox cars in the deep furrows that now etch my face. And, if someone focuses on my eyes, they will see what I call the cancer glint, a fleck of sadness embedded in the iris.

"I know you can beat this" is at best wishful thinking. There is no cure for the one hundred sixty or so types of cancer, and small cell lung cancer is not on the short list for marked improvements in survivability. As I told my unwitting accountant two years ago when he asked

7

about projected life spans for Ben and me in order to discuss some financial planning, "Everyone in Ben's family lives at least into their nineties. Me, my survivability is reassessed every three months." He didn't charge me for the phone conference.

4 THE TOUGHEST PART

There are so many downsides to cancer that it's not worth trying to list them all. If you need an instant shot of depression, just go online. I do find it helpful to read up on new advances and studies, but I go no further down the rabbit hole.

Two basic facts are etched in my soul: lung cancer is the deadliest form of cancer; and small cell lung cancer is the more rare and deadlier type. I now can deal with this reality. I am sick. I've got it—literally and figuratively.

What I cannot manage or sublimate is the impact this rotten disease has on those closest to me. To this day, my calm, capable husband Ben will be reading or watching a documentary with a cancer reference and the tears will silently stream down his face. My caregiving triumvirate, who came fearlessly marching in to help Ben and me during my treatments, rarely ask about my status. I convinced them, including my dear hypochondriac friend with a fascination for all things medical, that discussing the endless series of what-if scenarios and inconclusive test results is not helpful in my particular case. I hope that's easier for them. I know it's easier for me.

Buried deep down inside me is one of my two greatest fears. It's not death. It's a simple fact of human nature that continues to haunt me. As Anton Chekhov, who died of tuberculosis, wrote, "Whenever there is someone in a family who has long been ill, and hopelessly ill, there come painful moments when all timidly, secretly, at the bottom of their hearts long for his death." I don't want to be that someone.

5 DIAGNOSIS CANCER

February 8, 2010

It is an ordinary weekday morning. As I walk from my bedroom to the kitchen, I announce to Ben, "I am dying."

An attention grabber, I know, but that is not my intent. In fact, there is no intent. The words simply tumble out of my mouth. I am feeling fine, yet I know my statement is true.

March 19

The searing pain tearing across my upper back is not going away. This is not a symptom to be ignored. So, I call the office of my primary care physician and explain the pain is reminiscent of what I experienced when I had a pulmonary embolism eleven years earlier.

Even among the most dismissive of medical personnel, pulmonary embolism is not to be ignored. One hour later, at ten o'clock, I am with a nurse practitioner, then off for a ridiculous fee-for-service x-ray to see if I have a fracture before getting to the real diagnostic test—a CT scan.

By three o'clock that afternoon my doctor for the last seven years is personally on the phone to relay the results. That's the first give-away the news would not be good. In her typical, no intonation voice, she begins the very brief conversation.

"You have pneumonia."

"OK."

"The pneumonia is sitting beneath a five-centimeter mass in your upper right lung."

"That doesn't sound good."

"No, it isn't. It is very, very, very bad. I have called in prescriptions for an antibiotic and painkillers, and I've scheduled an appointment for you with a pulmonologist first thing Monday morning."

"Is this a doctor you actually know and recommend or is his name just on the top of your network referral list?" This remark is not as snide as it sounds. Prior referrals were less than optimal.

"I do know him. He's quite good. Here's the information."

That was the last I ever heard from the doctor I now refer to as my former primitive care provider.

Ben is standing near me during this conversation. Once I hang up, I relay the information. "Sure does sound like lung cancer."

"We're not going there. Right now all we know is there is pneumonia and a mass. Once we know more, then we can deal with whatever it may be."

That's my guy. We've been together for twenty-eight years and we have always been in sync when it comes to handling difficulties and crises. We stay calm, amass information, check sources and resources, devise a plan and work together to make it happen. Good thing we've had some practice. We'll really need it this time.

Our friend Mary Ellen is here from Boston for her annual three-week winter defrost. Lucky woman, she'll get to walk through this diagnosis process with us.

Fortunately, she and I have known each other since the age of thirteen when we were forced to carpool to an all girls' Catholic high school some ten miles from our hometown in the Boston suburbs.

March 22

The doe-eyed pulmonologist with the slight Lebanese accent sits knee-to-knee with me. All the while maintaining direct eye contact, he explains the CT scan done on March 19 revealed the mass sitting atop the pneumonia in my upper right lung is cancer. Grade on this test number one is an unequivocal F.

The bronchoscopy he would perform the next morning would allow him to determine if the mass is benign or malignant and, if the latter, the type of lung cancer.

He then outlines the possibilities. Basically, if it's non-small cell lung cancer, surgery may be an option. (In the relative world of cancer, this would be good news.) If small cell—the aggressive form affecting a mere fifteen percent of lung cancer victims—surgery would not be an option and the treatment protocol would depend on the stage of the cancer. Of course another test would be required for that.

"I know you cannot make any predictions until you have all the test data, but in general terms, I'm toast, right?"

For a full minute, Dr. Doe Eyes stares motionless at a blank wall.

"Are you familiar with this colloquial expression?" I ask.

He turns and looks directly at me. "Oh yes." He then returns to his silent contemplation of what exactly he should say to me.

At that point, it didn't matter what he might say. My mother died from small cell lung cancer in April 2006, four and a half years after she was diagnosed. It was a painful and ugly death.

March 23

At crack of dawn, Ben and I are at the local hospital waiting in the colonoscopy line. Obviously, no special treatment for us pulmonary patients. As I am lying in a rolling bed, watching a very nervous phlebotomist try to run an I.V. into my most delicate veins, a seasoned nurse stands at my feet and asks, "So what can we help you with today?"

"I'm here to see how long I have before I die."

Without skipping a beat, she replies, "OK, we can do that." Now this is a woman I can communicate with easily.

She wheels me down the corridor at a rapid clip and into her room. She preps me for the procedure, the whole time engaging me in an easy conversation. When I ask her about Dr. Doe Eyes she tells me she has worked with him nearly a dozen times and she believes he is a keeper. I am now breathing almost like a normal person. Within minutes of the doctor's arrival, I am asleep, the procedure is performed and I'm out of the hospital before lunch.

March 24

Ben and I meet with Dr. Doe Eyes. He confirms that the cancer is indeed malignant and it is small cell. An F on test number two.

March 26

My medical oncologist walks into the examining room, looks directly at me and says, "I'm so very sorry." That statement summarizes my diagnosis and prognosis.

This smart, quietly confident and direct man I dubbed Dr. Zen is my kind of specialist. He then begins the discussion of the ifs and whats. In short form, this is the story.

Small cell is the fastest moving and least common form of lung cancer. The results of the PET scan and MIR scheduled for Tuesday afternoon are key to staging the cancer and setting up treatment. Unlike most cancers that are rated in stages one to four, small cell lung cancer is so virulent it has only stages one and two. I'll have results no later than Thursday.

If the small cell cancer is still contained in the chest area, there is a twenty percent chance of living for five years, the benchmark for "surviving" cancer, if an aggressive combination of chemo and radiation are administered in combination over a period of about ten weeks, and are effective in reducing the tumor and forcing the cancer into remission. Clearly, a lot of ifs.

If the cancer has spread, the recommendation is to get a milder form of chemo for several weeks. That would temporarily shrink the tumor and increase "quality" of life for about three months. By month four, the show would be over. I would be toast.

Basically, every diagnostic test so far has had the worst possible result. So much for the luck of the Irish. However, the big test is next week. I really do need to pass this one.

As the shock of the initial diagnosis began to diminish, the reality of my survivability—or lack thereof—comes into sharp focus. It unplugs the governor in my brain that used to allow me to control outbursts—yelling, crying, screaming. Now, I cry unchecked. It's very disconcerting. I never was a crier.

The angry outbursts are a different thing. I have

long had a problem keeping my mouth shut when I feel someone or something is outrageous. As my friend Mary Ellen advised while riding shotgun in my convertible, "Please keep the top up on the car. Remember, you're not in Boston anymore. You now live in Florida where pick-up trucks have gun racks and the locals legally carry concealed weapons."

6 WRITING THERAPY

To help keep the hyper-emotional me in the background during the first six months of my cancer trek, I ask my closest friends to write texts, emails and yes, even snail-mail letters to communicate. It's not that I don't want to talk with them; it's the energy required to maintain a tear-free positive tone. Fortunately, I have pals who are funny, provocative and entertaining both in person and in writing.

March 29, 2010
Dear Phyllis,

I don't know how the hell you are managing. I keep trying to imagine, in my head, what each minute and hour are like and how you are coping. And what you might want, need or be able to use to get even ten minutes or maybe one hour or longer of just mental vacation from all of this. The prognosis is a little hopeful, right? Twenty percent is not horrible. OK, your luck on this one has royally sucked until now but it is definitely time for a turn around. I'm hanging on to the fact that (as your doctor said) aside from the f*#@ing tumor, you are healthy as Lance Armstrong. He did it. Others have done it. And you can too.

Huge hug,

Joanne

Afternoon Joanne,

There's no secret or magic about managing—there's simply no option. It's optimal to block this whole thing out of my head, but that's only an occasional occurrence. So, I just go with the unprompted bouts of crying and try to focus my attention on anything else. That too is easier said than done, as my powers of concentration have been minimized somewhat by the constant pain and the encroaching reality of what is happening.

The pain is less than it was a week ago, but the pneumonia is being kept in place by the tumor—nothing like one-upsmanship. After my Reiki treatment yesterday, I had several pain-free hours.

I'm having an usually sad day, so it's best to sign off now,

P

April 6, 2010

Phyllis,

Firstly, happy birthday. I reserve the right to re-celebrate your birthday in July. Where, I remind you, the horoscope sign is cancer. This must be like hair of the dog.

Hope you got the birthday video that we made for you. But mostly I hope that this passes quickly, that the side effects are not nearly as horrible as they warn, and that we are out by the pool hula hooping before you even

realize.
Lots of love,
Joanne

April 7, 2010
Dear Pam,

Now that's one exceptional birthday gift! The earrings are gorgeous and showcase my favorites—pearls and diamonds. You shouldn't have but they do look fabulous on moi!

I so enjoyed hearing about your trip during our call the other day. Sorry to make you cry. But since it is the "all about me" week, I am so glad to have shared this with you. It is a big help to my men and me, and I hope it will bring you good things to offset the bad.
Big hugs...

Dearest Phyllis,

I really am grateful that you are sharing this with me. I will not let you down. I'm quietly clearing my calendar, so I'm available ALL the time.

After I pulled myself together yesterday, I went to see my oncologist friend. When I told her the cancer was contained, she said you might have won "the lottery" for treatment of this type of cancer.
XO

May 5
Evening Mary Ellen,

Well, the truly shitty side effects have started. My twenty-four-hour weekly crash period now extends to forty-eight hours. And, as a surprise treat, it is followed by a teaser good day, only to revert to thoroughly wiped out for yet another day. Given the average life expectancy for small cell is so few months you can convert it to hours without using a calculator, these wipe-out hours are quickly racking up.

Plus, it does nothing for my complexion, which now resembles the color of wallpaper paste. If that isn't singularly bad enough, the old face is topped by a bald head all sitting above a chest emanating the same blotched glow as a slow-roasted pig. Where it not for my sunny disposition, I would look like complete crap. Thank the stars I bought those nine thousand dollar front teeth a few years back.

On the up side, Jake is resting more comfortably these days. He naps with me, so the dog now sleeps about eighteen hours a day. His latest trauma is the attack of the mockingbirds—think Hitchcock's *The Birds*. When Jake walks out the door, they start squawking and dive-bombing him. These nasty ass fliers must be protecting a nest or they are all off their meds.

So, person who reignited the Jane Austen art of correspondence, time to pick up your pen again. As Jane wrote to her sister Cassandra, "I have now attained the true art of letter-writing, which we are always told, is to express on paper exactly what one would say to the same person by word of mouth."

P

May 10, 2010
Good Afternoon,

Reading about the endurance test you are undergoing has hardened me. Every time some one starts to tell me about their breast cancer treatment, I find myself thinking, "wuss."

I can't wait to hear all those girlie secrets like, if you lose the hair on your head, do you lose the hair on your face? Like those perky whisker-like things on my chin and the hair over the lip fuzz? I just paid thirty dollars for a tube of Chanel lipstick that does not bleed into the vertical lines around my mouth.

So you're complaining about a sallow color? That's my natural complexion tone but with freckles that have grown up and are now called age spots.

Well, I'll be there on Saturday…This may sound insane, but I can't wait to get there. See you real soon. Speaking of which, I can see. I now have glasses with progressive lenses.

Stay strong,

Mary Ellen

7 TREATMENT IN REAL TIME

I decide the best way to keep the eight people who are my inner circle informed is to email out a weekly update entitled "It's All About Me." This eliminates any need they may feel to keep in constant contact and, most importantly, curtails the calls to Ben.

Despite the fact writing has been a central part of my life since editing Mrs. Demby's second grade class newspaper, writing this in real time is torturous. I type a sentence. I cry. I remember the day's events. I cry. I force myself to see the irony, humor or positivity in each occurrence. This borders on the impossible for me, the pragmatist, the person who values honesty at all costs and asks for it in return. However, I promised to do this for the great eight, and even though it takes me quadruple the time it should, I push on. It's the least I can do.

Round 1, April 5

Ben and I meet with the oncologist this morning to set up the chemo schedule. It is a three-month program:

three consecutive days (Tuesday through Thursday) for one week, then two weeks off. On Tuesdays and Wednesdays, the chemo is for about five hours. On Thursdays, it's two hours. It all starts tomorrow, April sixth, my sixtieth birthday.

As a special treat, I am getting an unusually strong drug on Tuesdays and Wednesdays, which accounts for the long treatment time. Because it often causes vomiting and nausea, I get to take a one hundred fifteen dollar pill to stem these effects before each treatment. Clearly, cancer is not for the uninsured.

Tonight at seven o'clock I get my first radiation zap. This will go on five days a week for six consecutive weeks. Each visit takes only ten to fifteen minutes. In exchange for the good schedule, radiation causes the worst side effects, which all the docs are saying start no later than the end of the third week and last throughout the remaining weeks before beginning to taper off. I won't bore you with all the potential side effects; suffice it to say I had to sign a document attesting to the fact I had been informed and then a witness had to sign as well.

Following my birthday chemo infusion, I head off with Ben for a second round of radiation. Fortunately, this should be the last evening appointment. I sit with three other women in the changing/waiting area. We all are decked out in shapeless exam gowns.

As the minutes drag by, one forty-ish woman begins a perky patter I learned to expect from patients decked out in all things pink. Sitting beside her is someone in her fifties, looking quite ill and explaining how debilitating nausea really is. The third woman, the oldest and frailest looking in the room, remains silent. Finally, a young male technician stands in the doorway and announces the machine is down, so we can all go home.

"Will it be repaired by tomorrow?" I ask.

"Should be."

"And if it's not, we all end up several days behind in our treatment protocol."

He nods. Aha! Finally, I have a focus for my subliminally raging anger.

"That's not good enough. The consistency of treatment is critical for me and I imagine for a lot of others. So what will you do? Send us off to another radiation center?"

"No, ma'am," we'll work weekends if need be."

"Why can't we use the other machine? It seems all your prostate patients are being treated tonight. Do you reserve the finicky machine for female patients?"

By now I'm rockin'. I'm ready for serious verbal combat. The tech looks increasingly pale. Before he can respond, the elderly lady walks over to stand beside me, facing the outnumbered tech.

"Well, young man, what about it? The inferior equipment is just for women?" The tech has a somewhat bemused look on his face. A rather odd reaction to the ongoing verbal assault he is so calmly enduring. Then he speaks. "Ma'am you're flashing me."

Sure enough, as the elderly woman was gearing up for battle the front of her johnny became untied. I could feel her embarrassment.

I turn to her and say, "Well, I never. What some people will do to get to the front of the zap line." As always, laughter changes the dynamic for the better.

Round 2, April 16

Physically, according to my oncologist Dr. Zen, I am doing "very well." In fact, during our weekly get-together on Tuesday, he reviews the labs and simply beams when he reads my white blood cell count (WBC)—a mere two-point drop after undergoing twelve hours of "aggressive" chemotherapy and six radiation treatments. My perfectly normal temperature, weight maintenance and pulse/oxygen level combined are merely afterglow.

As the honorable man he is, the doctor fully accepts responsibility for my chemo crash last Saturday. However, he is quick to add that one day of having every part of your body ache/burn/pulsate during the eight hours you are able to remain awake is about the norm.

By Monday, I feel the best I have since before the Ides of March. I start back exercising. Much to his chagrin, our dog Jake is my thirty-minute morning walk partner. This weekend, I'll add in water aerobics and that will be far more to his liking.

Monday afternoon, I have a quick visit with the radiation oncologist I call Dr. Zap. She and I actually spend more time checking out each other's shoes than my throat. That afternoon also ushers in a reasonable, reliable schedule at the Zapadrome. No more rescheduling due to malfunctioning equipment and no more after-dinner appointments. My zap tech Joe is a truly good guy who, like Dr. Zen, radiates (pun accidental) confidence.

On the agenda for next week—just a mere five days of radiation, two doctors' visits and one blood draw.

Among the many interesting side notes is radiation quickly turns one into a human Blood Hound. I can now accurately determine the toppings on a pizza— still enclosed in its cardboard container—at twenty feet.

Round 3, April 23

Week three starts off very well. I continue to feel good—just like a normal person. Then comes my Tuesday morning appointment with Dr. Zen.

My white blood cell count tanked—from eleven last week to 1.5 For the uninitiated, 1.5 equals an "F", as is fail or f*#@ed. For the initiated among you, I cannot get the shot that helps boost my WBC due to the daily radiation regime.

The doctor tells me this WBC knockout is completely normal (these cancer folks have a very odd definition of normal) as it has been two weeks after the first chemo treatment. This is when the WBC reaches its nadir. So, for the ensuing five days I remain on antibiotics and house bound, except to go the Zapadrome daily. Ergo, I must stay healthy because for the time being I have virtually no immunity.

According to my wise doctor, my WBC count will increase by next week so I can continue the chemotherapy. Who would have ever imagined wanting to get infused with toxins, one of which is in the same family as mustard gas?

True to prediction, on the very same day, tingling started at the top of my head. This is not a giggle feeling, more like angry ants racing across the crown of your head. It doesn't last long, but it means the molting has started. So far, no gobs of hair have dropped off, but I'm expecting to whip out Ben's electric razor next week. I've decided to go with a buzz cut.

I wrap up my all things medical week with a quick visit to Dr. Zap. The radiation chick is at an apparent loss as she listens to my response to her initial question: "How are you feeling?" I tell her I feel fine, no sore throat, no cough, no skin burn or rash (although the zaps have peeled off a few layers at the radiation site, which is the size of a quarter), no headaches, no problem sleeping. I exercise daily and continue to eat like a wild boar.

Again, according to the written predictions of

when patients will definitely feel rotten (documents provided by both the chemo and radiation practitioners), a rather distasteful array of radiation side effects were to be underway by now. Realizing I was losing her interest and throwing off the statistical accuracy of the side effects onset, I concede that I do succumb to afternoon fatigue. This helps.

Round 4, April 30

Following the now typical Saturday crash day, week four begins exceedingly well. Ben and I spend Sunday planting fifty shrubs and flowers around a new palm tree. Then, we did some pruning—specifically, my hair.

The most striking thing about being bald is when I slightly extend the tips of my long, pointed ears, I look just like Yoda. This is not self-deprecation; it's fact. Every time I remove my hat, tug on my ears and ask, "Who do I look like?" the answer is Yoda.

Fortunately for Ben and me, my sister Pamela arrives from San Francisco Sunday night. All has been arranged in advance, knowing despite my lack of grace in accepting help, we are going to need it over the next several weeks.

Monday signals the start of the second and final double-dose week—five consecutive days of zaps capped with twelve hours of chemo over three consecutive days. Cancer treatment in real time is not for the faint of heart.

My next hurdle is to pass the WBC test on Tuesday, allowing me the privilege of being infused with more toxins. I did—from 1.5 to four. The four of us in the examining room —Dr. Zen, Nurse Linda, Ben and me— all started to laugh. (Trust me, you can only understand this reaction if you were physically present.)

With all the lab results solid and me feeling great, Dr. Zen wants to know what I am doing, as it is atypical to be in good shape at this halfway point in the treatment. In addition to following all his and Dr. Zap's instructions, I exercise daily (except crash days) and have almost daily Reiki sessions with my personal Reiki master (aka Ben).

Very attuned to my "no surprises" rule, the good doctor reminds me that even though I am sailing through week four, weeks five and six will be bad, as in very bad. The chemo/zap crash will be longer, it will take longer for my system to recoup, I'll have to go back on antibiotics and stay very close to home. Fair enough. The up side is that the six-week radiation gig ends on May seventeenth and I can then get a single shot to accelerate my WBC growth.

We then swap a few funny stories before Dr. Zen remarks how nice it was to have such a short visit. As he is leaving, he grins and says, "May I have a hug?" This sweet man deserves a win.

The following day, the amazement at my statistically aberrant good health continues. Dr. Zap goes through the weekly roster of questions before leaning forward and saying with absolute sincerity, "Really, please do tell me what you are doing." She then asks me to tell her more about Reiki. Perhaps I am inadvertently laying the groundwork for a new career for my nuclear engineer/energy consultant Ben?

Week 5, May 7

This week ushers in some long-predicted and wholly unwelcome side effects. Sunday afternoon signaled the end of the weekend crash, which had lasted forty-eight hours. However, Monday sucks from beginning to end. It is the very first day I simply did not have the strength to get out of bed. I am chauffeured to the Zapadrome and then promptly plunked back into bed. After my treatment, Tech Joe informs me I have thirteen more zaps to go— three more than initially discussed with Dr. Zap.

To most bystanders, a mere ten percent increase may not sound like a lot, but to a weary, pale, goal-focused woman, this is monumentally disconcerting. And, the fun continues into the night when I awake feeling as though the red ant army is doing practice drills on my chest. I soon learn this is radiation dermatitis.

Tuesday with Dr. Zen is delightful as always. All labs are fine and he quickly admits the 6.5 WBC is completely unexpected and unexplained, but he is "glad to take it." Ben then whips out his multi-dimensional color graph of my weekly WBCs and the boys get immersed in a game of show me yours and I'll show you mine.

Wednesday, Ben and I meet with Dr. Zap. Seems the compulsively detailed doc had forgotten to explain thirty zaps is actually my goal, but the (and I quote) "bonus round" is thirty-three. The absolute minimum for efficacy in my case is twenty-eight. OK, but if I am able to go to thirty-three, that means week six will be another chemo/zap combo. Hard to fathom this is the actual "prize" for completing the bonus round.

On the up side, my strength rebounds on Tuesday and continues. The morning water aerobics is energizing as is the always-divine Reiki. Plus, after two failed tries, I have an ointment that makes the radiation burn tolerable, albeit still most visually unpleasant.

Not surprisingly, I am hungry and must move on to my fourth meal of the day.

Week 6, May 14

This week is one of unrealized predictions—almost. The ominous, major crash precipitated by the cumulative impact of twenty-four max dosage zaps and six high-octane chemo treatments is nearly a complete no-show. Even the predictable weekend downtime never occurs. Tuesday is a very low energy day, but in the world of side effects, this barely counts.

Tuesday also is the weekly meeting with Dr. Zen and Nurse Linda. The labs for this, the nadir week, are relatively solid—with the all-important WBC coming in at a totally respectable two. Once again, temperature, weight and blood pressure all hold steady. As a reward, I get to take a pass on the typical five-day antibiotics regime. My heavily taxed digestive system is most grateful.

No visit with the dynamic medical duo is complete without some laughter. When Dr. Zen enters the room, he flashes a broad smile and says, "Good to see you." I reply, "Really?" He nods his head and says, "I wish you would come every day. You make me smile." Gotta love this man.

I subsequently notice the very perceptive Nurse Linda intensely staring at me. "Is something wrong?" I seem to have startled her a bit. "No, there's nothing wrong. It's just that you are doing so well."

As the visit is ending, Dr. Zen reminds me to stay close to home and not get sick, as my immunity is very low. I look him in the eye and announce, "I will not get sick." He chuckles and replies, "Ok, I know that look. You will not get sick. Fine."

The laughter continues through to my Wednesday brief check-in with Dr. Zap. She's clearly taken note of my boringly consistent good health. This week she walks in wearing another pair of kick ass heels and says, "Doing fine?" When I answer in the affirmative, she laughs, "Of course you are."

She then asks about the medication she had prescribed the preceding week. This is a standard drug used to coat the throat as it becomes more constricted—and often dotted with ulcers—as the radiation treatments advance. Although my swallowing capabilities are only mildly impacted, I had asked for the prescription so that I would have it on hand when needed. I told her that I have not needed to take it yet. Again she replies, "Of course."

She confirms the remaining zaps and I again reiterate my "out" clause once I reach the goal of thirty on Monday. She nods and then adds, "But, of course, you will be able to do thirty-three."

The visit is about to end when Dr. Zap reminds me about the ten prophylactic cranial irradiation (PCI) treatments that are recommended if the upcoming MIR and CT scan show the cancer has not spread. This is a precautionary, optional treatment prompted by the fact the next target area of small cell lung cancer is typically the brain. As I tell her, this is a ways off and quite conditional, so I prefer to defer spending time researching and discussing this right now. I feel it's much more beneficial at this point to focus on finishing this treatment marathon and planning our trip to Rome and the Amalfi Coast. Agenda item tabled for now.

I awake this morning feeling tired and cheated. This is supposed to be the last day of radiation. Besides, the skin encircling the aptly named target area is now continually burning (fortunately at varying temperatures) and beginning to flake off. The cure for this feeling is food and sleep. I did both before trekking off to the Zapadrome. Now after a milkshake, quiche and bread, I'm back to what passes for fine these days.

Weeks 7 & 8, May 21 & 28

Week 7 is supposed to be celebratory, marking the end of daily zaps and the completion of three of the four scheduled chemo treatments. Both goals are met on May twentieth, but at an unexpectedly high physical and psychological cost.

The week starts out well. Mary Ellen flies in and we all have a laid-back Sunday. After the Monday zap, Mary Ellen and I spend a whole two hours trawling through two funky boutiques. Remember, for someone who has been absolutely nowhere except doctors' offices and treatment centers since March 19, this is a major outing.

Prior to the start of chemo on Tuesday, Ben and I meet with Dr. Zen and Nurse Linda. The labs are good—all systems go for chemo. And, for the first time, I am eligible for a Neulasta shot on Saturday, which should boost my white blood cell regeneration. Dr. Zen says there is no need to see him next week; just come in for a quick blood test. He reminds me that the following two treatment-free weeks will give me an opportunity to rest and recuperate.

Even though my man Joe is on vacation all week, his trusty colleague Laurie is in charge of my remaining zaps. Because the start time and duration of my chemo treatments vary, I call thirty minutes before the chemo ends to get a zap time. Like Joe, Laurie does everything possible to get me in quickly—and Tuesday is no exception.

For the very first time the Wednesday chemo treatment starts off quite poorly—I have to wait thirty minutes before the assigned nurse begins telling me what is wrong with every single vein in both arms. This is knowledge I already have. The chemo has corroded my always-delicate veins.

Nurse Negative then ties a tourniquet and adds a blood pressure cuff to pump up a vein. She succeeds only in numbing my hand and causing acute pain. When she walks away to get a heating pad, I ask Ben to go to the front desk and request another nurse to start the line. There is just too much bad Karma.

A second nurse appears and within a few minutes has me laughing and a line inserted. However, Nurse Negative is still responsible for hanging my multiple meds and is never in sight when the buzzer goes off to change out one of the five bags hanging from my I.V. pole. So, the entire process takes four and a half long hours.

Fortunately, the zap folks are able to take me at two-thirty and I could see Dr. Zap just before the appointed time. Her focus is entirely on scheduling prophylactic cranial irradiation in July. This washing of the entire brain with radiation is recommended for contained small cell cancer patients if, after the radiation/chemo protocol is completed, there is no evidence of cancer in the body or the brain. The tests needed to make this determination are a CT and a ghastly MIR, which are typically done six weeks or more after the chemo is completed.

PCI is a three-week, daily process. My custom-made *Man in the Iron Mask* headgear is placed over my face and bolted to the metal table. For about fifteen minutes gamma radiation is lasered into every part of my brain. The available efficacy data are from a study of patients with limited stage small cell lung cancer diagnosed between 1989 and 1997. Of the less than ten percent receiving PCI, the five-year survival rate was thirty-four percent (versus twenty-eight percent for those not undergoing PCI). If this is not enough of a teaser to sign on, there is a paucity of data on the neurological impacts, but absolute certainty that your hair won't begin to grow back for three to four months. With all these happy thoughts swirling within my bald head, I amble off for zap thirty-two.

Fortunately, chemo on Thursday—the ninety-minute treatment—goes very well. However, as Laurie is off, the zap tech delays my scheduled twelve-thirty appointment for thirty minutes. So, I head home for an hour before going to the Zapadrome for my final appearance. Once there, I sit for another half hour until another tech comes out and says there is a delay. Suffice it to say, the built-up anticipation of ending this day of pain and horror explodes. Sounding like Maggie Smith minus the British accent I pointedly inform the young tech that people like me, who measure their future in three-month intervals, jealously protect every minute. Sitting on a stiff chair in a cold waiting area is not living.

Foolishly, I think Friday will signal the start of feeling better—consecutive days without medical treatments, abatement of side effects, regaining strength. Instead, on Friday afternoon, I trundle off to bed to rest. A mere seven days later I am able to get up.

So Week 8 draws to a close. Among the sadistic, nefarious characteristics of cancer are both the disease and the treatment reward best efforts with debilitating physical and psychological effects. Perhaps that's why the medical community speaks in terms of survival, rather than cures.

Weeks 9 & 10, June 4 & 11

Week 9 is the gradual rebuilding of strength, shaking off anemia, a blood test and a visit with Dr. Zen.

The half-hour discussion focuses on PCI. The short version is that Dr. Zen, Dr. Zap, Nurse Linda and Ben all feel it should be done, assuming the MIR does not show evidence of brain cancer. (In that case, the decision would be whether to move from "prophylactic" to "intensive" cranial irradiation.) I appreciate the consensus of opinion, which is consistent with published research, but I'll be the only one on that cold metal table covered in a neck to top of head mask as my entire brain (which I have grown to appreciate, quirks and misfiring synapses notwithstanding) is zapped.

The only heretofore unknown is if, after receiving the PCI, there is no evidence of brain cancer for two years, there is very little likelihood that it would occur at all. The same cannot be said for cancer in other parts of the body.

After the visit, the schedule is set for an MRI (this time with anti-anxiety medication taken beforehand) on July sixth and a CT that same week. The PCI would start around July twenty-second and continue for fifteen consecutive days. The guess is that it would then take about two and a half weeks to recover.

It's now the end of week ten and the end of the initial treatment regime. Thirty-three zaps, twelve rounds of chemo, sixteen doctors' visits, twelve blood draws, one bronchoscopy, one CT, one MIR, one PET scan, one set of tattoos, one radiation fitting, two Neulasta shots.

Reportedly, it should take two to three weeks to recover from this final round of chemo toxin infusions. However, as Dr. Zen replies when I ask if I will ever feel fine again, "It is possible, but age impacts the ability to return to what you regard as normal."

This last day of chemo is a terrific day on every

single level. First thing, I am presented with a luxurious graduation gift and a very special card. Then, off to chemo with some well-deserved treats for the team.

Working with "my people" (the crew on this week is Pamela and Ben), the chemo front desk angels, Liz and Tammy, have their wish granted—a long visit with Jake. Then, the chemo team is presented with a lavish and creative fruit bonanza highlighted by dolphins sculpted from bananas. I can wholeheartedly praise this creation, as my involvement was wisely restricted to cutting up one pineapple and providing an unneeded level of commentary. All twelve then receive a gift certificate to a neighboring spa. I couldn't think of any group more deserving.

As the I.V. comes out of my arm for the last time, the spectacular chemo nurses and schedulers gather around to sing their own rousing rendition of "You Will Survive." Odd as it may sound, the lyrics sung by these incredible women simply make you want to get up and dance.

Pamela, Ben and I then go out to celebrate by buying me a wig (which despite all my preconceptions actually does not look fake and weird, it just feels fake and weird) and having lunch. The day is capped off by a most excellent dinner and new signature dessert.

And, so it is. The final edition of this weekly update.

8 THE RECOUP

I am glad to have ended the weekly emails. I am dreading what's coming next. I doubt I could manage a positive tone and my confidants don't deserve to be confronted with all that.

It's now a week since my last round of chemo. The best guess among the medical folks is this crash should be not as bad as the weeklong collapse I experienced after ending the radiation treatments and the third round of chemo on the same day last month. Hoping for less awful—how inspiring.

As it turns out, predictions are just that. The level of pain is somewhat less as the internal and external chest burns have diminished noticeably over the four weeks since my last zap session. The physical pain and debilitating exhaustion remain strong. Most crippling is the psychological devastation.

In anything resembling a normal set of circumstances, I should be feeling physically better every day, getting stronger, feeling more positive about my life and how long it just may last. I'm not.

Every time I wake up, whether from a nap or a night's sleep, my first thought is "I have cancer." My next thought is "Why get up?"

It's hard to find reasons, even just one. I will never have my life—the life I created—back again. Cancer has already taken so much that is irretrievable. I can never even trick myself into believing that I am an independent person who is fully prepared to take care of herself.

Despite the fact that I am not a reality TV contestant, I have been labeled a survivor. Real survivors are those heroic people who endured the ultimate cruelties inflicted by war, racial discrimination, ethnic hatred and other forms of barbarism. Me, I am just another person who contracted an incurable disease.

This sounds so self-pitying because it is. But, it is not just the ramblings ignited by depression so common in Little C Club members. It is based on a host of simple facts.

1. Once I heard my diagnosis of small cell lung cancer, I knew I would never return to "normal." I continue to learn to live with what now passes for normal.
2. Being able to say I am cured of cancer is simply delusional. The best I can hope for is a determination of "no evidence of disease" for an extended period of time and being among the seventy-five percent of cancer survivors who do not experience multiple cancers— recurrences and/or different types of cancer.
3. Profound fatigue is a side effect of both chemo and radiation. Although I was told this subsides after several weeks, it can last for years. I'm now at year three…and counting.

4. Like many chemo patients, I experienced tinnitus, the annoying and persistent ringing in my ears. As Nurse Linda assured me, this is normally a temporary condition. In fact, the condition persisted in only two of her patients over the past ten years. Meet patient number three.

The most far-reaching of these cancer realities is most people do not want to know how you are. The question is merely a conversational courtesy. I know now not to answer it honestly. However, I assume my doctors will be an exception. Bad assumption.

On Monday, eleven days after my last chemo treatment and thirty-two days after my final zap, I meet with Dr. Zap for a follow-up visit.

At the reception desk I am asked to sign a form once again swearing my insurance has not changed and telling me that I owe them some nine hundred dollars. Fortunately, Ben carries a three-inch thick binder to all appointments. It includes a running spreadsheet of all invoices and payments along with all my test results, medications and other salient information. This shows that I already paid the invoice—another one in the ten thousand dollars to date out-of-pocket costs I am personally responsible for under the expensive and extensive health insurance policy I also personally pay for each and every month.

Dr. Zap walks in thirty minutes late for the appointment, sits down without apology or explanation and asks how I am. So I tell her in rapid-fire detail about the debilitating fatigue, the throat constrictions, the sporadic burning inside my chest. No doubt, my fury and frustration about being told all side effects should be over in a few weeks after the last zap and yet I am still feeling ghastly is evident in my tone.

She takes umbrage, saying I am angry and directing it at her. Good god, why would she take this personally? Of course I'm angry. Who the hell wouldn't be angry? I'm angry that what I was told and what I am experiencing are two different realities. I am angry that asking questions and questioning approaches are viewed as somehow ungrateful—after all, shouldn't I be grateful there is at least a treatment protocol that can be attempted in my case?

I allow her to do the maternalistic "given your anger and focus on quality of life issues, it is best not to have any further discussion of the PCI now. This can all be delayed."

I respond by telling her although the timing may not be optimal, it is imperative to me that a preliminary schedule be set for the PCI and specific questions answered today. So, for the first time, I hear the shop of horrors menu. This is the recitation of the permanent cognitive impacts, the increased incidence of cataracts, the extreme fatigue that can persist for months, and all manner of other forms of scary ugly. And, to ensure I never again will have a reason to say that predictions fail to match reality, she adds that even if the PCI is effective and no brain metastases appear, I could of course develop cancer at any time in my liver, lung or other major organ.

To sum it all up, I ask Dr. Zap if she agrees that doing PCI is a crapshoot. She replies, "Yes."

When we get in the car to go home, I notice Ben looks unusually stressed. "What's wrong?"

His voice cracks and tears run down his face.

"Everything we are told is always so very negative." We drive home in silence.

The next day is an early morning appointment with Dr. Zen. He reviews my blood work, listens to a brief recitation of how I am feeling and says that I should be feeling much better shortly. All very matter of fact. He asks if I have made a decision on the PCI and listens for a brief period to my questions and concerns before saying most of this is in Dr. Zap's area and I should speak further with her. He then—for the first time ever—looks at his watch and says as he walks out the exam room door, "Well, I have to keep moving along." Don't we all.

9 FUGGEDABOUTIT

I follow Dr. Zen's lead, deciding to adopt a dismissive approach to my cancer. I avoid it, circumvent it, relegate it to the very back of my brain. Medically, I cannot make it go away. But I sure can get it the hell out of the way so I can live what's left of my life.

As always, I let my innermost circle in on my plan.

Dear Utmost Support Team,

After much, much ado, I've come to a decision on how to move forward. Since you four create the treasured support/assistance/encouragement network, I think you'll understand and appreciate this decision.

The approach, which I dubbed fuggedaboutit, is disinterest in all things cancer related.

Over the past several months, I have learned some simple truths that have shaped this approach.

- Cancer is an ugly and cruel disease that is never really cured.
- Once treatment ends, doctors have no active involvement/interest beyond ordering

regularly scheduled screening tests to look for reoccurrence/new cancers.

- The diagnosis and treatment have rendered me physically debilitated and psychologically diminished. Although incremental improvement is possible, side effects are permanent and a return to "normal" is a fiction.
- No one enjoys being around sick people and constant talk of illness is depressing.
- My first thought when I wake and my last thought before sleep cannot continue to be "I have cancer."

This approach is predicated on the expectation the MIR and CT on July sixth show no metastases in either my brain or elsewhere in my body. I then will have ten consecutive prophylactic cranial irradiation (PCI) treatments in mid July to reduce the probability of developing brain cancer and then spend four to six weeks recovering. The last cancer thing will be a PET scan sometime in September.

Given this schedule I should be back to what is euphemistically called a "new normal" in early to mid September. At this point, my normalcy may/will include:

- groveling for some last-minute contract assignments before the moneymaking season ends;
- flying to upstate New York to attend Joanne and Ray's somewhat annual Labor Day bash;
- spending several days in October at the Ringling International Arts Festival with Pamela;
- visiting my much-loved, cancer-stricken, soon-to-die (from what else but lung cancer) aunt in Phoenix;

- attending a niece's wedding in Albuquerque in late October;
- welcoming Mary Ellen as a Florida resident in November; and
- decorating the house to the max for Christmas.

To get this whole approach kick-started, Ben and I leave tomorrow for the Ritz in Naples where I will spend two days in the spa having all the toxins accumulated over the past three months scrubbed off my virtually hairless body.

10 BRAIN ZAPPING

Unlike my earlier proclivity to flunk every diagnostic test, I passed both the MIR and CT scan in July, enabling me to undergo Prophylactic Cranial Irradiation (PCI). Not so lucky me.

Getting up close and personal with cancer, chemotherapy, thoracic radiation and death roils up a lot of negatives. Absent from this long list was terror until I underwent PCI.

First, I am fitted for a mask, a series of cross bars covering the top of the head down to the neck. This is a short procedure, painless but frightening. I asked the techs to take photos of me in my mask, locked down on the table. I thought seeing the photos would allay my fears. Wrong again.

Prior to each treatment, I lay down on a cold metal table, a tech puts the mask on me and bolts it to the table. The alignment is checked and the tech leaves the room. I am now alone in a cold dark room with a laser pointed at my head. A disembodied voice tells me to lie still. The short zaps begin. As they continue for several minutes, I tell myself not to move, barely breathe, suppress the horror pulsating inside me.

Each of the ten days I undergo this treatment I tell the tech on duty that I am terrified. This is not hyperbole. This is fact. All I can think of is potential disasters. There's a power surge and the laser controls are frozen. The tech monitoring the process has a heart attack and the laser is left to its own devices. I sneeze and the zap obliterates a vital part of my brain.

Each of the three-member tech team tries to help. I'd met them all during my thoracic treatment days when I appeared a lot more light-hearted. One gives me a quick French lesson before the zaps begin. Another comments on my outfits. The third keeps telling me this is all good. I value their kindness, but it doesn't wipe away the terror.

After the last brain zap, the tech team comes into the treatment room and presents me with my mask. I know these men are being sweet, but I cringe when I take the mask.

11 GOOD, BAD, MAYBE BUT NEVER FOR SURE

As any respectable doctor will tell you, medicine is an art. It is by no means a definitive science. That realization cuts two ways.

Prior to my brain zapping, the tests showed no metastases. The mass in my right lung was reduced by half and is most likely scar tissue from the thoracic radiation. A few months after the PCI is completed, my oncologist decides to do a CT scan. This shows a further fifty percent reduction in the mass, "suggesting a positive therapeutic response" and, best of all, "no findings to suggest progressive or new disease." This is happy dance time.

Refusing to let any cancer mar my Christmas, I insist upon delaying the next CT scan until the start of 2011. Good thinking. This one shows the mass is stable, but there is a pleural effusion (excess fluid that accumulates between the fluid-filled space surrounding the lungs).

The next CT scan is in June. This one shows the mass is stable in size, but pleural thickening has developed in two other areas of the lung. The recommendation is for another test in three months to exclude active metastatic disease. In English, this means the cancer may be on the move again.

The CT is repeated in September and "suggests" a worsening of the pleural thickening in two locations, both deemed "suspicious" for pleural malignancy. The recommendation is for a PET/CT.

The roller coaster of test results continues. The CT in January 2012 shows a stable condition, with no suspicious findings for active malignancy/metastases. Score one for the home team. I decide to take another six-month break from all tests.

The June CT raises the possibility of malignancy in the pleural thickening. Then again, it could just be getting larger. No one knows. So, the oncologist orders a PET/CT for September.

I am rescued from this cascade of "what ifs" and "no one can say definitively" by none other than my insurance company. Since the initial diagnosis, I have had no issues with my health insurer. Amazing, but true. The insurer refuses to authorize the PET/CT unless I first undergo another CT scan, a bone scan and an ultrasound. Patently ridiculous from a medical perspective and totally out of the realm of possibility for me. I simply won't do it. I didn't.

At this point, no one can say anything to make me change my mind. Even if I did the PET/CT, there would be no conclusive answers. If there were evidence of cancer in the lining of my right lung, I would have to have a lung biopsy. Then the only treatment would be watered down chemo (an oxymoron?). That would be trading two months of illness for an extra two months of life—maybe. If it's not cancer, and the fluid keeps building, I may have to have the fluid removed. I can wait to find out about that one.

So the treatment cycle ends, mercifully. The stress of so much testing, the physical drain of receiving twenty-nine times the average annual radiation dose a nuclear plant worker receives—or the equivalent of twenty-nine years of normal background radiation we all receive—and the tortuous days waiting for results are over. Enough already. If the lung cancer goes on a rampage, the pain will alert me. No need for advance notice.

12 SAYING GOODBYE

There was one other person I wanted to tell about my illness, but I couldn't. Some three months before my diagnosis, my uncle died quickly, peacefully in his recliner while watching a poker match on TV. His wife walked into the living room and found him. She was the sick one— emphysema, lung cancer, pancreatic cancer and a host of chronic illnesses that kept her essentially homebound and tethered to an oxygen tank.

My aunt began radiation in March 2011, just a few weeks before I started my regiment. I called her regularly, being sure I sounded strong and clear on the phone. When I couldn't muster the energy, I wrote her letters. She was enduring a lot of pain because she felt it would be too difficult for her beloved granddaughters to lose both grandparents in such a short period of time.

"I'm ready to die," she told me. "I've lived long enough. But I want to last for maybe a year, for the girls."

We talked over the course of several months, but the elephant—why I hadn't flown out to see her—was always in the room. Finally, in an unguarded moment I started to explain how sorry I was for not being there for her. The uncontrollable sobbing started. Ben took the phone from me. I could hear him affirming, "Yes, she is very sick."

When I took back the phone she said, "I knew it. It's lung cancer, right? Oh shit." That made three of us in less than five years—my mother, her sister (my aunt) and me.

We both started to laugh. "No wonder you knew so much about the side effects of radiation, you smart ass. You were in treatment the same time as me."

She asked how I was dealing with it all and I told her it was manageable except for a single thought I could not get out of my head. I told her about walking into my kitchen in February and telling Ben I was dying.

My aunt's intuitive abilities were fierce. When I told her my fear she immediately said in her imitable fashion, "Oh for chrissakes, that was not a prediction. That was a premonition, telling you to be prepared for what was coming at you. Trust me, you will make it. I won't."

As soon as I was cleared to fly, Ben and I went to visit. She was pencil thin and frail. However, that didn't stop her. Actually, I could not remember anything that could stop her once she made up her mind. She had coffee for us when we arrived and food ready for lunch. She had invited her son and daughter to drop by, but only after we spent several hours together laughing, telling old stories and updating one another. We had a great day, but by early evening it was clear her energy was depleted.

The next morning, my aunt, her daughter, Ben

and I went to visit my uncle's grave. It was good to chat with my uncle for a while and I know he got a kick out of the token we left on his gravestone—a golf ball. My aunt then insisted on taking us all to lunch before returning to her condo.

Once settled in, Ben and I sat with her for a few hours. She adored Ben and she loved me. As we stood at the doorway to leave, my aunt said, "The only thing I'm going to miss is seeing you again."

I held her close. "Oh you will see me. I am planning on visits from you as soon as you get settled. I love you."

She died four months later—a few days shy of the one year she had wanted. I miss her.

13 CARPE DIEM

Big Cities

For as long as I can remember, my motto has been "when the going gets tough, go on vacation." So we did—a lot. And, we continue to travel to places we want to explore.

What better way to launch the travel schedule than a somewhat spontaneous jaunt to Paris in January 2011. Pamela was already slated to be there, Mary Ellen had never been to the City of Lights, I needed a serious change of scenery and Ben needed some alone time.

We stayed in a charming bed and breakfast across from Notre Dame. The location was ideal for walking and provided easy access to the Paris Métro. Each day we went exploring. We took a walking tour of Le Marais, strolled through Île Saint-Louis, Canal Saint-Martin and Rue de Passy; visited Musée d'Orsay, La Louvre, Musée Nissim de Camondo and Centre Pompidou; and toured Opéra de Paris Garnier.

What I had not anticipated was the oppressive fatigue that overpowered me late each afternoon. For the prior ten months, I was always with Ben who would take charge while I recouped. Now it was up to me to take care of me. It was terribly important I meet the challenge.

Most days I did fine, but whenever some little thing was amiss, I began to melt down. No patience, no calm, just annoyance with myself for not being able to control myself and rectify the situation. And, as I later learned, both Pamela and Mary Ellen were watching closely, knowing they should not interfere, but wanting to help. Wisely, they did not intervene.

Some six weeks later I flew to New York City to enjoy some real theater and Chinese food with Joanne. We walked, shopped, dined, partied, fully enjoying a real girls' long weekend. This brief trip assured me I was ready to travel.

Big Country

Ben and I decided to see a good chunk of America the old-fashioned way—by car. We hit the road in early May heading to California.

My idea of a long car ride is four hours. Jake averages around three hours. Fortunately, Ben loves driving for hours on end through some of the most catatonically boring landscapes this country has to offer. I give you northwest Florida, central Texas, Kansas, Missouri.

Long road trips can be made more tolerable by casual motel sex with hot quiet guys (a la *Thelma & Louise*), drug-induced hazes worthy of Hunter Thompson or the adoption of Ben's perspective—from Sarasota to Palm Springs were the miles traveled to get to the start of the road trip. So, during these scenic-free miles, Jake and I shared a lounge chair mat in the back of the Jeep. If I moved too much, Jake would hop in the front and ride shotgun for a few hours. When the dog had had enough for the day he would jump into the driver's seat when Ben got out to fill up with gas and wouldn't move to let Ben get behind the wheel.

After two and a half days of coma inducing, non-stop driving, the scenery became enchanting. The landscape across the southern swath of New Mexico and Arizona is remarkably similar—majestic and hard. The striations in the rock faces vary greatly, each revealing the manner of its creation. The sprawling wind farms in Arizona and California become contemporary sculptures set across spare ridges and desert floors. The dramatic shapes in motion do create a special beauty and I could see Ben embracing the landscape with his mind and his soul. It gave him peace and a sense of calm I had not seen in a long while.

Eateries along major interstates are typically not enticing. However, there are lucky moments. Ours was at lunchtime in Deming, New Mexico. A staff member at a local winery shop recommended La Fonda (no relationship to the famous hotel in Santa Fe). This was a roadside cafe along a one-lane dusty road (beginning to sound like a country western tune, ey ya?) serving the best chicken enchiladas we've ever tasted. Our waitress personally makes the fabulous taco chips at her house each morning and gave me the recipe. This was a true taste of America.

The minute we hit Cambria our vacation began. A lovely town on the coast, a welcoming country inn, a dog-friendly beach, great food, fun shopping and gracious locals. We arranged for a private pet sitter for Jake as we took tours of the Hearst Castle in neighboring San Simeon, an amazing hilltop architectural wonder that merits more visits. Among the many fascinating facts is the 165-room vacation home was designed and built between 1919 and 1942 by the groundbreaking woman architect Julia Morgan who, among countless other achievements, was the first female graduate of Ecole des Beaux-Arts in Paris, introduced steel-reinforced concrete buildings to San Francisco, and designed and built a total of seven hundred structures.

Not far up the coast is another wonder—an elephant seal rookery. We pulled into the parking lot, walked along the planked perimeter of the beach and there below laid thousands of elephant seals. During this time of the year only the three thousand-pound females are molting, flipping sand, scratching with their five-fingered fins and generally lolling about while their young spar with one another and conclude their thirty days of learning how to swim and survive on their own. The males had already mated and, not surprisingly, shirked all parenting responsibility and headed off to Alaska.

The next highlight was Carmel. Despite the breath-taking wealth of this seaside community, the landscape and architecture are subdued, the people are engaging and often throwbacks to the early '70s in speech and perspective. Needless to say, the restaurants and cafes are wonderful and the shopping is affordably sublime.

After some three thousand or so miles (I found it best not to actually count), we pulled into San Francisco. What a pleasure (at least for us) to pile into Pamela's apartment and not have to get back into the Jeep anytime soon.

Both Ben and I love this diverse, vibrant, walkable, beautiful city rife with energy, personality and fantastic food. There's espresso to drink when sitting at outdoor cafes in North Beach, browsing through Chinatown and Japantown, strolling Union Street and the flower market, buying freshly baked bread at the Ferry Building's Saturday market, enjoying the beauty of the Japanese Garden and Golden Gate Park, and gazing at the breathtaking views and architecture that regularly pop into your sightline. For a slice of SF camp, we went to see the outrageous and long-running *Beach Blanket Babylon*. And for theatrical majesty, we drove to Berkeley to see the National Theatre Live presentation of *Frankenstein*, arguably the best play I have ever seen either live or on film.

The real highlight of San Francisco was the opportunity to enjoy the city with Pamela. She loves her town and we loved being there with her. And, despite having two adults and one dog who cannot understand why he can't sleep wherever he wants, our hostess did not toss us out earlier than planned.

We hit the road east on May 26 bound for an overnight stay at Yosemite. As a first time visitor I was duly impressed by the natural grandeur of the park. It was one Ansel Adams photograph after another being brought to life just for you—especially at Yosemite Falls. Despite all the posted info about bears, I saw neither Yogi nor Boo Boo, just a lot of Bambi's relatives way too accustomed to humans.

My beloved, born on a mesa top Ben decided to drive east from Yosemite via Sonora Pass. As we climbed ninety-five hundred feet into the cloud covered sky, the temperature dropped some thirty degrees, the lush green landscape became snow covered and the narrow mountain road with fifteen percent grades regularly disappeared as we switch-backed up the sliver of roadway. This spectacle induced a for-real panic attack. After the literally breath-taking drive, even Ben admitted that he had never driven such a death spiral road in the mountains of New Mexico or Colorado.

Blessedly, the landscape flattened and my breathing returned to normal for a few minutes before we came to screeching halt behind a flock of sheep being herded down the right lane of the highway. Welcome to Nevada's Loneliest Road. Yes, that is the real name of the aptly named byway. If you simply awoke and found yourself traveling this patch of pavement, you could easily assume you had been transported to another planet. With raindrops dotting the windshield as we drove along this eerie moonscape, it was easy to see pointillism in motion as I tried to guess the type of vehicle approaching from the opposite direction. You'd be amazed at how long it takes for those first orange dots against a gray fog to coalesce into an orange semi tractor-trailer.

The next day we meandered through Arches National Park in Utah. The landscape here is so reminiscent of New Mexico with its towering red rock formations looming above a desert-like floor. Perhaps best known for the Balance Rock (its name tells the story), it is a serene yet haunting place.

That night we began the push home. We zipped through Colorado, Kansas, Missouri, Tennessee, Kentucky, Georgia and northern Florida stopping only for gas, an occasional lunch and a place to sleep for those four nights.

When we arrived home in June, we had racked up some seven thousand miles, spent long hours in quiet conversation, and seen the spectacular and the ordinary in seventeen states. This is indeed a remarkable country of contrasts and commonalities. And, of course, quirks.

The topographic monotony of Kansas is only interrupted by the profusion of pro-life road signs.

I have absolutely no idea what Tennessee looks like as its highways are densely lined with tall trees.

The Santa Fe River is in Florida.

Roma

Before embarking on our long-awaited trip to Rome, each member of the triumvirate came to visit us—Joanne in August, Mary Ellen in September, Pamela in October. This schedule was ideal. I did some part-time work on what turned out to be the last of forty-nine ballot question campaigns I worked on during my career. And, it allowed me and Ben to rest up between visits and thoroughly enjoy each one.

In mid-November we jetted off to Rome, a city we had put at the top of our "must see" list. Our centrally located hotel—just two blocks from the Pantheon—allowed us to easily walk to most of the architectural and historic jewels housed in this ancient city. We had no set agenda for our two-week stay, beyond going to Naples and Pompeii for two days. We left our hotel each morning and embraced the city, its sights and each other.

Allowing our energy levels to dictate the extent of sightseeing was key to fully enjoying the Eternal City, aka the City of Love. Being there together, walking the cobblestone streets with our hands intertwined convinced me that neither appellation is completely accurate. For us, it should be the City of Eternal Love.

We toured the exquisite Doria Pamphili Gallery and Apartments, strolled through the ruins of the Forum and the majestic Coliseum, walked up Palatine Hill to visit the Augustus Caesar house. In Vatican City we absorbed the splendor of the Vatican Museum, the Sistine Chapel and St. Peter's Basilica. We climbed Michelangelo's Grand Staircase to Capitol Hill where we visited Capitoline Museums. We often walked by the Victor Emmanuel Monument, the glorious white marble wedding cake structure that dominates Piazza Venezia. After viewing the art in the Borghese Gallery, we rented a motorized bicycled and rode throughout the luscious gardens on a perfect Sunday afternoon. We window-shopped along Via V. Veneto and the Spanish Steps. Longing for a taste of the old USA, we had our first ever hamburger at the Hard Rock Cafe.

We traveled by train to Naples and aimlessly walked around the port city, stopping for a world-famous pizza. The following morning we took a short train ride to Pompeii. Despite its history of devastation, there is a singular dignity and beauty to the ruins and corpses frozen in time and place. For some inexplicable reason, I found it comforting.

We appropriately devoted our last day in Rome to churches, small ancient places set a bit outside the main parts of the city. We climbed the Holy Stairs and sat silently in Basilica of Saint John Lateran. It was a wonderfully calming day in a bustling city, and the perfect conclusion to our trip.

Alaska

The forty-ninth state had long been on our "must see" list. We just figured we would do the more physically demanding trips before we hopped on a cruise ship. So much for long-range planning.

We flew into Vancouver in late June and enjoyed a few days walking around this gorgeous and welcoming city. Then we boarded the ship and set off along the Inland Passage.

I was not thrilled about this trip, but Ben was eager to see the wildlife and the mountains. He more than earned it.

Despite my skepticism, Ben had booked a land excursion a day. It took barely a day for me to get rid of any hesitation and embrace this adventure. Besides, who would have guessed Alaskans actually dress visitors for success when exploring this majestic and magical place.

Leaving Ketchikan to climb trails opening on to spectacular views of Tongass National Park in a specially modified Tomcar adventure kart called for screaming yellow or army green high waders with matching jackets. To emphasize the challenge of navigating narrow, rutted logging trails, the ensemble was topped by a motorcycle helmet in gleaming silver. After spending several hours racing through mud holes, each outfit took on a slick brown patina.

With Ben behind the wheel and me strapped in beside him, I saw the sheer cliff off to his right and a slightly less treacherous drop to the left. Normally, I would have voiced my trepidation and warnings to drive carefully—as if someone could on the muddy, rutted path. Instead, I thought of the headline "Couple flies out of

Tomcar and tumbles to their death in Alaska." Miles better than "Yet another woman in Florida dies of lung cancer." I turned to Ben and yelled, "Let 'er rip."

He pressed the accelerator to the floor to climb each hill and kept it there as we splashed into the mud and it rained down on us. I could not stop giggling—I mean giggling like a five year-old. Playing in the mud washed away the inhibitions of adulthood.

Still clad in our high waders and slickers, we tramped through the world's second largest rain forest. Here the summer weather forecast was rain with a chance of clouds and partial sunshine followed by rain.

To get an up close and personal look at the Mendenhall Glacier, Ben bought us $2.95 modified plastic shower curtains. They kept us dry while reducing the wind impact on this summer day.

When it comes to style, no one and nothing surpasses the classic styling of orcas. The sleek black contrasted against dazzling white shows why they justly deserve the title of killer whales. The orcas and other majestic marine life—humpback whales, otters, seals— captivated us for hours as we sailed in the chilly, windy and frequently rainy environment. The normal triple layering approach proved insufficient, so we wrapped towels around our heads, secured them with baseball caps and encased ourselves in deck blankets. Our eye-catching on-deck ensembles had passengers requesting to photograph us.

The fun continued the next day with a hike along a small portion of the historic Chilkoot Trail, traversed by Klondike gold rush prospectors. Even our brief climb made it clear why Nordstrom became a retail giant.

Realizing he couldn't complete the trek, he set up shop along the trail repairing boots. Today's hikers don jeans, hiking shoes, two layers of shirts, a lightweight winter jacket and baseball cap for the cool and rainy summer hike.

At the end of our trail, we popped on a safety orange life jacket and slipped into a pair of Wellies. We were set for rafting on Skagway's Talya River. There was no need to wear a swimsuit under our three layers of clothing. In July, the water temp is an unwelcoming thirty-eight degrees.

For our last tour, no one gave a hoot about what the humans were wearing. It was all about the two- to eight-week old Alaskan husky pups raised here in Denali by the best all-time musher and multiple Iditarod winner Jeff King. As we stepped off the mini-bus we were each handed a puppy to cuddle. This interaction with adoring tourists helps socialize the little guys prior to beginning their racing careers. Needless to say, we were delighted to help.

At each stop along this journey, we were introduced to new people, animals, landscapes. We sensed our place in this harsh, expansive, daunting environment. Like Pompeii, Alaska displayed the brutality and the serenity of living and dying. Most importantly, the Alaskan adventure triggered the release of long stifled giggling and good old-fashioned fun. When we boarded our flight home, we took this spirit—ridiculously dubbed "posi"—with us.

Philadelphia

We hadn't visited the City of Brotherly Love for more than a decade. The opening of the Barnes prompted the return visit. The works by some of the greatest European and American masters of impressionism, post-impressionist and early modern art are outstanding and displayed as they had been in the home of the collector, Dr. Albert C. Barnes. The city is also home to the Rodin Museum, a small but striking Beaux-Arts building housing one of the most comprehensive collections of work outside Paris by one of the world's most renowned sculptors.

The immersion in art was balanced by a strong dose of American history. We visited Freedom Hall, the Liberty Bell and several historic parks and homes. The visit also prompted a mini reunion. Joanne and her husband drove in from New York and Joanne's brother, whom I have known for more than forty years, came in from the Philadelphia suburbs. We spent two nights at dinner laughing and recounting stories from our college days in Boston. Once again, I realized time spent with good friends is an invaluable treasure.

Hawaii

The offer from Pamela was irresistible. Two weeks at an oceanfront condo in Oahu. Off we went in January 2013.

Pamela met us at the airport, placing leis around our necks as she said aloha. In the Hawaiian language, aloha means affection, peace, compassion and mercy. During our stay, we experienced all the meanings of this welcoming word.

The delightful native docent at Plantation Village told us endearing stories of the Portuguese, Japanese and Chinese sugar cane workers who lived in this humble community in the early twentieth century. During our tour, she made mention of certain implements and other items that had "gone missing" in recent months. The Village could not afford security and a group of homeless people was camped just outside the perimeter. Although it was more than reasonable to assume who the thieves were, the elderly docent merely noted what was missing and hoped one day the items would be returned.

Doris Duke's island home is a perfect contrast to the Plantation Village. The contemporary house, adorned with Islamic art, is perched at the water's edge providing a breathtaking panoramic view of the ocean and mountains. Set to one side of the house is a swimming pool and bathhouse, which Miss Duke called her playhouse. Ben nicknamed it Daisy Duke's pool house. The estate makes it clear that money has its privileges. However, in the aloha spirit, all beaches are public, so beneath the Duke home locals and visitors regularly gather for a day at the beach.

One of the natives taking advantage of the beach in front of our condo was a pregnant monk seal appropriately, but inelegantly, named Rock. Early each morning, volunteers cordoned off the area Rock had selected to rest for eight to ten hours that day. A volunteer stood guard, making sure that no visitor crossed into her space. These are not helicopter volunteers, they are conservationists helping to educate visitors about the urgent need to protect the Hawaiian monk seal, one of two remaining monk seal species.

The natural hush of the verdant Waimea Valley Gardens created a calming spirit that followed us as we strolled through this historical, cultural, botanical and ecological haven. Visually we became one with the landscape—or a senior take on an Anne Geddes baby photo—by poking our heads through the enormous leaves.

Ben and I flew to the Big Island to visit Volcano National Park in the town aptly named Volcano. We began with a tour of the park led by a young national park employee we dubbed Ranger Runny Nose. Poor thing was allergic to carbon dioxide. Unfortunately for this interesting and entertaining young man, the volcano was burping out dangerously high levels of the noxious gas into the environs.

Ben expected to see volcanic activity, but that was not to happen. He did see amazing fog, steam and the red glow of the carbon dioxide emissions rising above a large tract of moonscape. Neither we nor Mark Twain were bothered by the gas. According to the plaque commemorating the humorist's visit, "The smell of sulfur is strong, but not unpleasant to a sinner."

Next up was a drive to Kona, an area featuring lush hillsides, lavish homes, beachfront lodgings, aromatic coffee plantations, the understated Hulihe's Palace and the recreated City of Refuge. The ever polite and respectful Ben managed to tee off a rather hulking interpreter by barraging him with questions. Apparently, this native Hawaiian was there to demonstrate the art of making fish lines and hooks, not to discuss it.

After returning to Oahu, we ventured out to Pearl Harbor. The stark beauty of the harbor and resounding impact of respectful silence were all encompassing. There are no words to describe standing above the sunken USS Arizona, the resting place of eleven hundred and seventy-seven sailors and marines killed on December seventh.

Since the infamous day in 1941, more shipmates have joined their brothers. Upon their deaths, USS Arizona survivors can be interred in the sunken vessel.

In between morning beach walks and lazy dinners, we visited a number of sights including the North Shore surfing haven, Waikiki Beach, Chinatown, Diamond Head and the Royal Hawaiian.

Throughout the islands we encountered welcoming people, marveled at majestic whales, gazed at painted sunsets, toured poignant and historic venues, and absorbed the landscapes that pose for the camera. We experienced the fullness of aloha—affection, peace, compassion and mercy. It's an enchanting island way of life.

Commonalities

These trips made it imminently clear that the most memorable moments are those created with others. My traveling companions are close friends. We enjoy one another as much—and sometimes more—than the places we are visiting. The people encountered add to the interest and fun. A silly moment, an interesting conversation, a provocative dinner discussion create a unique memory safely packed before heading home. This is living.

14 PSYCHICS

Among the many transformative moments over these past three years were conversations with three psychics. The first was a fifteen-minute reading, more for fun than anything else. The woman told me she felt powerful healing around me. I attributed that to Ben and Reiki.

The second was a telephone session given to me by a friend as a birthday gift. The friend had a long association with the psychic, but had provided no details about me. Unlike any other reading I have ever had, this woman pressed me for specific health details before telling me she did not see death.

The third psychic took my breath away. As I was walking into her room, the petite Vietnamese woman looked up and made two statements. "You are psychic. You no longer have cancer." She proceeded to touch upon a number of subjects with laser accuracy and to recommend I continue to travel so that I could continue to teach those I meet along the way.

Before leaving she spoke of the one dominant fear

I had carried with me over a three-year period and had never mentioned to anyone—not even Ben. "Don't worry," she said, "you will have a peaceful death at the end of your long life."

I could actually feel a weight dissolving. I had never been afraid of dying but I was terrified of dying badly. Not anymore.

15 IF I WERE YOU...

Clearly, I am not you. I do not purport to know you or how you think. However, a number of people have asked me to write down things they should say and do when a friend or loved one is diagnosed with cancer. So, I am obliging with great trepidation. For those who are sick, we are all as individual as our cancers. For the support teams, bring the real you to the party. That said, here are my thoughts.

No blaming. People get cancer because they do. Leave it at that. What's past is passed. Move along.

Laugh. Cancer can grow exponentially in the absence of humor. That's my belief and experience. The sheer weight of the whole disease/treatment/dying thing can be staggering and more often than not induces depression. So watch comedies, tell jokes, search out the humor even in the most sobering of situations, do silly things. Laughter is more effective than antidepressants, plus it's free and it's freeing.

Truth only. This applies to the c person, and the

friends and family. When asked a question, answer truthfully. Skip the BS, the spin, the niceties. Don't duck and cover. Just answer the damn question.

No waterfalls. Cleaning out the tear ducts is fine, but cascades are not. If you must completely fall apart— and sometimes that is exactly what you need to do—don't drag other folks along. Lock yourself in the bathroom, go for a walk, stick your head in the freezer (this last one is my personal favorite). Most importantly, absolutely no one looks attractive when bawling.

Don't ask; won't tell. If you need to know how your friend or loved one is faring, ask. If you don't ask, most won't tell because no one likes being around a whiner—even when the whining is more than justified— and talking about virtually anything other than cancer is typically a welcomed relief for everyone.

It's all about (*fill in the blank*). Some days, it's all about the patient. Some days, it's all about the spouse, parent, partner, friend. It's never all about a work associate, casual acquaintance or Facebook friend.

Ask not what you can do for the patient, JFDI. (For those of you who have never worked in a nuclear environment: Just f*#@ing do it.) Any self-respecting sick person is extremely unlikely to ask others to do what really needs to be done. I give you ironing, laundry, food shopping, weeding, dusting, cooking, mopping and most other mundane chores of daily existence. Just make a meal and deliver it to the house. Don't call first. Don't come into the house. Just hand it to whoever answers the door. Send flowers. Write a letter. Drop off a funny DVD. Drive your mower over and cut the lawn.

Ask the c person to help you. Once the patient

is feeling better, ask her to do something for you—help rearrange a room, fix something around the house, shop for the perfect dress, assemble a slide show. We all need to be needed. We all need purpose.

Keep in touch. But keep it reasonable. Do not inundate the person with phone calls, emails, texts, Tweets. Initially the person will be overwhelmed with attention. Within a few months, the peripheral people will have fallen by the wayside. The cancer will still be there.

Exercise. This applies to everyone. Pick up your own good self and walk, swim, bike, lift weights, do Nia, yoga, hip hop abs, Pilates or Zumba. It doesn't matter what you do, JFDI. It's great for your mind and body.

Do advance work in advance. If you up and die on your loved ones, they will be saddened. If you do this before completing your pre-death chores, they have every right to be royally pissed at you. Make sure you have a health care directive and a will, discussed palliative care with your local hospice, and expressed your au revoir/ciaio/hasta luego wishes to a responsible friend or family member. Do this before you are too sick to make the best decisions.

Live. Grab onto life and live every day as best as you can. And, regularly say "I love you" to those you love. This is one time repetition is encouraged and appreciated.

16 PURPOSE

For me, the best way to fuggedaboutit is to focus on someone or something in need of assistance. After all, as a friend advised me, it's all relative. However miserable it may be for me at a given point in time, there's always someone somewhere who is far worse off. Of course, such altruism is not omnipresent; there are minutes, hours and days when I succumb and declare myself the singularly most put upon, unlucky person in the cosmos.

When a neighbor broke her left wrist on the day after I was diagnosed (she had broken the right wrist a few weeks earlier), I showed up with a basket of snacks, chopped fruit and straws. I fluffed her pillows, straightened her quilt and coaxed her to try to sleep. She felt better and so did I.

Another neighbor developed bronchitis. As befitting a sick male, he was in bed, moaning and complaining. So I made my outstanding chicken soup and delivered it to his house with a note saying, "eat this and be cured." He later swore the soup really did do the trick.

Our godchild Sam was beginning high school in Massachusetts. She is a good student but seems to lack a real understanding of college—from how to select the right school to admission processes and financial aid. So I organized a field trip to Boston for Sam, her mother (my niece), my sister and Ben. We arranged tours at our alma maters and hotel rooms for us all. My hope was to mix some good time together with a gentle push for her to begin to prepare for her future. I knew this was at least a year premature, but I didn't know if I would be around in another year. So, better soon than never.

I was arranging a get together with a couple in their mid seventies. Like me, the woman was sick of going out to dinner. I suggested bowling. The four of us were relatively well matched—we all sucked and we all laughed our way through two games.

At least once a week, I nestle my bare feet in the white quartz sand of Siesta Beach, look out into the blue waters of the Gulf and begin to move to the music. This is Nia, a sensory-based movement program drawn from the martial, dance and healing arts. My instructor, who holds three other jobs, didn't have time to publicize her classes in the area newspapers. I did.

When the older sister of two neighbors was diagnosed with lung cancer, they invited me to coffee to have a frank talk with the three of them. All were in their eighties and the patient seemed unflustered about it all. As she said, "We all have to die from something." However, her son was about to undergo his first round of chemo that day. He was very nervous and she asked me to speak with him on the phone.

"Hi Robert. This is Phyllis, the neighborhood

cancer go-to girl. I understand you are joining the chemo crowd today."

He laughed a bit when he said yes.

"Are you afraid?"

"Yes."

"Phew. That's a relief. If you weren't afraid I'd have to tell your mother that there is something really wrong with you."

"Really?"

"Absolutely. All of us are afraid. But the good news is that thinking about it is the worst part. If you can keep your ass in a chair for several hours without going stir crazy, chemo is no big deal."

As the conversation continued, he laughed more and he laughed louder. Now he was ready for chemo.

17 BEAUTY TIPS & TRIALS

Cancer is fattening. Yup, I even confirmed it with my oncologist. Most people receiving chemo gain about ten pounds. Those sneaky doses of steroids do the trick.

When steroids are mixed with I.V. infused drugs, the complexion takes on a rosy, natural looking glow for two days. Personally, I'd rather just buy blusher.

Radiation and/or chemo stopped me from perspiring under my arms and the top of my head. (I had so much of both, it was impossible to determine which was doing what.)

Undergoing treatment does save a great deal on personal maintenance. During the first year, I had no outlays for haircuts, hair dye, deodorant, olive oil soaps, eyebrow waxing and pedicures. Had I been on a higher personal care level, I also could have foregone lip, chin and bikini waxing, perfume and scented body creams.

Essentially, my personal care demands were akin to those of a Sphynx, the breed of hairless cats. Additional similarities are a full, round abdomen (aka pot belly) and sagging skin around the jowls, derriere and stomach.

I do have a well-shaped head and look good in hats. That not withstanding, a sixty year-old bald woman sporting a jaunty, flattering hat still is viewed as a cancer patient, not a fashionista. Then, there's the unmistakable look in strangers' eyes—fear, pity or a combination of the two. None is a good vibe to communicate to the bald lady.

18 LITTLE C MOMENTS

A woman well into her Social Security days sat waiting to be called in for her radiation treatment. She smiled and I inquired, "How are you today?" She responded, "Well, not too great. I got past breast cancer a few years back and now I have cervical cancer. At least with this cancer, I get tingling sensations in places I barely recall having."

After giving me the full diagnosis and prognosis, Dr. Zen brightened up. "You are really in excellent health." Ben, Nurse Linda and I all looked askance at one another. Dr. Zen took note. With a sheepish smile, he added, "Well, except of course for the cancer."

I asked a chemo nurse if there was a specific name for the I.V. poles from which the bags of drugs are hung. "No, just poles," she replied. "In fact, if any of us should lose our job, our training and experience qualifies us for a second career as pole dancers."

I asked my aunt about the side effects she was experiencing from radiation. "Besides being exhausted, not much. But then again, I am virtually bionic. Every morning

I put on my wig, snap in my false teeth and turn on my hearing aids. There's not much left to destroy."

My hair stylist went to visit a friend who, a year earlier, had been diagnosed with pancreatic cancer and told he had four to six months to live. When the stylist next saw his friend he casually remarked, "You look good for someone who has been dead for six months."

A friend sent an email recently to confirm a lunch date. It had been several months since we had seen one another. She signed off by writing, "Thanks for sticking around."

19 THE BACK STORIES

Mary Ellen, The High School Friend
March 19, 2013

You were here with us when we first got the diagnosis. What was your reaction?

It was denial. I said to myself, "This isn't happening."

So, as Sarah Palin would ask, how's that denial thing workin' for ya?

It's working well. It was easiest to deny it when I was here with you and Ben. I could repress the cancer reality, but I couldn't see how you could. So for me to start dwelling on it around you was going to do absolutely nothing positive. As Brian Williams said, "Confronting the rude is depleting to your health." It was harder when I was at home, reading your emails and letters.

Did you think about what you would do and say when you got here?

I decided to just be normal around you. I couldn't come down and morph into a super helpful house manager; that would have been out of character. For example, why would I come here and cook dinner? I never do that. Cleaning the bathroom, washing dishes, making cookies were all things I do.

When you came down again in May, the radiation was over and almost all the chemo. Were you prepared to see the aftermath?

Ben explained on the way from the airport that you had no immunity so he asked that as soon as I got to the house to take a shower. But I told Ben you had to see the outfit I had on as I wore it just for you. So Ben said he'd take a photo and show you. When we got to your house, you did stand at your bedroom door and checked out the outfit.

How did I look to you?

When you were bald, I liked your look. It was sort of alien, fragile. You did Yoda well. I wasn't shocked when I saw you. You looked different, but good. My rational mind accepted the change, my emotional mind didn't.

Did you see the cancer glint in my eye?

I didn't see sickness, but I saw fragility—a look I had never seen before in the forty-nine years I've known you.

How did Ben react to you when this all began?

He gave me a non-touch hug. That's how we do it. And I said to him, "You're her best friend now." He was the center, the core for you and for me.

Did you ever feel guilty or bad for yourself?

That's my upbringing. If you don't feel guilt, you are bad. There were moments when I was back home, I would start thinking about my life if you weren't still on this earth. You are the most important person to me in the physical world. So I was feeling very bad for myself. And then I said to myself, "What the f*#@ is wrong with you?"

Did you ever feel helpless?

When we were in Paris in January 2011 you had a terrible day. And I could see it. I knew you needed to do this trip, you had to do it. Yet I didn't know how to help you.

Do you think I'm going to make it?

Yes, I always have. I see it in you. I saw it just the other day.

Pamela, The Sister Friend
March 26, 2013

When I called you on April 5, 2010 to tell you about the cancer and ask you to fly here to help, what was your initial reaction?

It filled me with sadness immediately. It felt like that sadness literally filled up my body. As I listened to what you were asking me to do, I realized I would keep that sadness to myself because it wouldn't be any great comfort or support for you. I had to go into a different way of feeling and thinking until I got off the phone with you.

Were you able to process what I was telling you?

Pretty much so because I clicked into help mode. Short term, I can provide help. So I really listened very hard and almost went into a work mind set, so I could really focus. The emotional side of it I could focus on afterwards. After I hung up, I just couldn't stop crying.

Shortly before you first came here, you sent an email saying I've been packed for two days and sitting here, now what am I going to do?

If I had had my way, I just would have thrown some things in a bag and flown down there. But that's not what you wanted, and it's very important to listen. Most of the time people will tell you what they want and you are certainly one of those people. It was difficult for me to stay at home and wait to come.

Was it easier to be here?

Yes, I was on-site and there were things I could do. Sitting back and waiting is extremely difficult for me. So I cancelled everything on my calendar and waited until the date you wanted me to come down.

There are wonderful lessons to learn in all of this for both of us. Asking for help is very difficult for both of us. It must be something to do with the way we were brought up. This is an opportunity to learn on both sides about asking and receiving.

It was clear to me when you called that you had a plan. I needed to make sure I could accommodate the plan.

We established something very important in that phone call. We reconfirmed candor. That was very important to me to be to be able to speak clearly. We made a deal that we could ask each other anything and get an honest answer. I can't say I always asked all my questions, but the ones that I asked, I knew you'd be very straight forward with me. Second-guessing in this environment would be very destructive. I couldn't have operated in that way.

What did you not ask me?

There were times I wanted to ask more clinical things and to ask about contingency plans. One thing I never talked with you about is death. Instead, I started reading. I've gone through a whole reading list on death over the last few years. You getting this disease is a completely different experience for me than Mom or our aunt (both of whom died from lung cancer) or any of the friends I have lost. I keep trying to find a way to work through this and to be supportive and make sure I'm listening when I should be listening—especially when you say you don't want something.

I don't tiptoe around you anymore. I did at first. The first two weeks I came, I just went to bed every night and cried. Then one morning you came in and you hugged me. You started to cry. Something changed then for me. Some degree of acceptance started to creep into who I am. That's when I took over the ironing, which I never do, the laundry, the vacuuming. I realized for right now that was all I could do. I could take over. It was almost as much for Ben as for you because Ben so desperately needed to be relieved of the household chores he was doing so he could focus on you one hundred percent.

Where you surprised when I called you and asked you to come here?

No. I knew we had been rebuilding our friendship since Mom died. I wasn't surprised. I was very pleased that you called. I would have been surprised—and devastated—if you hadn't because I felt that Ben, you and I were at a point that if something like this, or anything, came up you could call me.

What was the hardest time for you during those first few months when I was in treatment?

The first time I went to chemo with you. I found it disconcerting walking into this bright, sunny place with so many people there and the excellent nursing staff running around. I thought it was rather a light-hearted approach. I realized afterward that it's really a very healthy approach.

Hadn't you been to chemo before?

I had with a friend. But then I almost ran out of the room screaming. My friend later told me she was just watching me and even though I said all the right things, she saw how much pain I was in. So finally she said she needed a huge favor. She asked me to go pick up her car from the dealership. It's interesting how we take care of each other in these circumstances.

Did you notice any changes in my personality over these past three years?

I can't remember seeing you in a single instance where you did anything out of character. I see differences in your mind set from when you first started chronicling things and you had me read some of what you wrote. I found them so full of anger. I remember saying you have to give the reader a break here because no one will be able to read this. It is so full of anger and rage. And you said you were angry and asked if I was. I said no, I'm sad. One of the things you said very early on was that you wanted to find a way to do this with grace. And I've seen you do that — to get through the anger, to put boundaries around what works for you.

Was there a turning point?

You said I could ask you anything I wanted, but other than that you didn't want to talk about your illness much anymore. I thought that was a major turning point for you. For you to put this in a place and move along with your life. As you said, this allows you to get out in front or beside the cancer and to never be behind it again.

What the funniest or happiest moment?

To me this has been such a process of learning and growing. This has changed me and has surprised me how much it has changed me. Suddenly, I started thinking about you as my little sister. I think that moment when I was first at your house for a few days and you hugged me and we had a little cry. That was an important moment for me emotionally. It allowed me to go forward.

Do you think I'll make it?

This is a very difficult question and I don't know how to answer. I think there is a finite time, so my answer is "no." I want to be wrong.

I talked a lot with my oncologist friend about small cell lung cancer and the prognosis. She hoped I wouldn't go all positive on you. So I think I'm a grounding point for you.

Over the past three years I have had to find a path, a way to live with this. Together, we do fun things, we travel. This has allowed me to understand living in the moment.

Joanne, The College Roommate
May 1, 2013

When I called you and told you the diagnosis, what was your first response?

My first response was please make this a nightmare. This is not happening. Oh no. This can't be happening. It can't be true. Classic denial. At the same time, there was this sense that kicked in and said, "Phyllis can beat this."

We've reached this point in the history of cancer that when you hear "cancer" you don't necessarily think death right away—even when it's a bad form of cancer. You hear lots of stories of people who have cancer and they are OK. At the same time I am listening to you and hoping that I am having a nightmare, and I'm going to wake up and this won't be true. I'm also thinking, "It's Phyllis, right? She's an ox. She's a bull. She's a titan. A little bit of cancer, that can't hurt her. "

One of my main take-aways from the conversation was the story you told me about when the doctor was very serious about telling you what you had and you said, "You mean I'm toast, right?" I hung on to that. Maybe this won't be a nightmare. Maybe this will be real. Maybe Phyllis is a kick-ass titan who can deal with it. But no matter what else, this is yet another opportunity for comedy.

Haven't you found that many stages of this saga have been comedic?

You're funny, so as a remedial strategy it works.

I've always been a fan of the Norman Cousins approach of laughing it away. Even though it's a myth, I like it.

When you came down to visit were you surprised by anything?

Yes, I was surprised, but in the most positive way. I was awe struck. I thought you had the most amazing attitude. You can't imagine what it does for people around you. It's not fair that you have to hold up everyone around you, but as my former boss used to say to me all the time, "Life is not fair." Your determination and approach to keep this out of your life, to not let it control you is what everyone around you needs.

What else could I have done? I never thought there was an option.

Many people do not have that reaction. People react across the spectrum. Some people shrivel up and just give in. Other people fight like hell. The rest do something in between.

What were some of the other funny moments?

It was fun going wig shopping. I never knew you'd look good as a redhead. And I loved that photo of you and Ben sitting on either side of Jake. He was facing the camera with his paws hanging over the back of the couch and the two of you faced the opposite direction so all anyone could see were two bald heads on either side of this furry dog.

How did I carry my baldness?

You carried it quite well.

Did you ever want to run away from it all and just say I don't want to deal with this anymore?

No, not for a second.

Did my diagnosis have any impact on your health perspective?

Because I'm a hypochondriac and a neurotic, I expect bad things to happen. So I wouldn't say you getting cancer changed the way I think about illness. Although, and this is really selfish, it means a lot to me that you have stood up and adopted the attitude you did. I remember talking with Ben early on and Ben was also focused. He said, "We're going to fight this. You can't think it's going to win. You have to win." For me, it makes me have the illusion of feeling stronger. If you're stronger, I'm stronger by association.

It's kind of a positive thing. I am very aware that when it comes to thinking about the negative side of your diagnosis, my brain shuts down. I'm not going there. Ben isn't going there. Phyllis isn't going there. So why should I go there?

Do you think I will make it?

Of course I do. Absolutely.

Ben, The Husband/Reiki Master
March 20, 2013

**When I was first diagnosed we came back home,
stood in the living room, cried, hugged each other
and you said in my ear, "The doctors will do their
best, but I will heal you." All I asked was how?**

The night before I woke from a sound sleep and
realized I would learn Reiki. For some reason I had studied
and read about the practice years earlier. It just came to me
that this is what I could do to help you.

I contacted a Reiki master the following week but
her class had started a month earlier and they were halfway
through the course. She could hear in my voice the
importance and immediacy of my request. The day I had
to start my training was your birthday and your first day of
chemo. You said I had to go, even though I didn't want to.
But I knew we both had to do what we had to do. You
needed to go to treatment alone and I needed to do this
class.

**Do you have any fond memories of being in the
chemo room with me?**

Of course. We were sitting next to an elderly
woman who was clearly frightened. Every time the nurse
tried to start the I.V. line, she jerked her hand away. You
suggested I hold her hand. So I moved over to sit next to
her and said, "You look like someone who needs her hand
held." Immediately, the lady began to talk. I could feel her
relax. And before she knew it, the nurse had completed
her task.

Then there was the morning that you got a sharp pain in your forehead. You asked me to make it go away. I got up, placed my hands on your head and within a few minutes you said it was gone. Watching this was an elderly chemo veteran sitting across from us. He looked at us as if we were voodoo practitioners.

Like most people, you started to do a great deal of online research. Was there anything positive you found?

In the early days of the treatment, I'd get up in the middle of the night worrying and researching small cell lung cancer. Finally, I got to the point where there was no value in researching anymore. I wasn't learning anything new or much that was positive. However, that didn't undermine my confidence in us. You were going through treatment in amazing fashion and keeping everyone's spirits up. It was a hard balance. We both were putting on a brave face. In private, I would cry.

How did you regain your balance after hearing the diagnosis?

Once I realized I could help, the sadness, anger, helplessness mostly ended. I focused on recovery and health. My belief was shaken though during the fifteen prophylactic cranial irradiation treatments. I knew I just had to give one hand to you and the other to Reiki. That anchored me.

How did you view the visits of the triumvirate?

When each one flew in, as I drove to the airport, I'd make a list of things they should know before seeing you. I didn't want to scare them, but I wanted them to know how you looked, felt and what was going on. I knew they were probably having a more difficult time than I was because I was here. They were left to their imaginations, to wonder. Knowing they are good, strong, loving friends, I knew it was going to be difficult. It was interesting to watch them cope.

Pamela had to be in action. For a break, she would drive over to the gourmet food store and buy exotic oils and vinegars. After her first two-week visit we ended up with at least a one-year supply. Joanne came in with her usual bravado, but it was easy to see it was a façade. Mary Ellen, who was here during the diagnosis process, was clearly shaken to the bone.

Did they talk with you about how you were doing or how they were doing?

No. It was pretty easy to read on our faces. The emotions were pretty evident. Each one was holding their deep emotions in check and maintaining a good front. My relief when they were here came from their ability to engage you in conversation and make you laugh.

You have always been the anchor in my life, and during this period of time, you were still holding that position. But whenever I looked at you, my heart would break. My greatest sadness was watching you. What I needed was to be sure you were OK. Did they help?

They each offered to be there if I wanted to talk or if you needed anything. I offered them the same in return. But the only person I really talk with is you.

Was it more helpful to have people here?

It wasn't better or worse. It was different, quieter when they weren't here in July and August. By then, though, the effects of all the treatments, especially the PCI, really hit. We were in recovery mode. There was a lot of sleeping, resting. That's where Jake came in to help us both.

What was the singularly worst moment in the past three years for you?

The day we got the definitive results on the PET scan and MRI. That's when it hit. We were driving home and the call came in from Nurse Linda who read the pathology report to us.

What was the best moment in the past three years?

There were a lot of different ones. The general comfort I got from doing the Reiki and how it helped give you control and comfort was the vehicle for keeping me focused. Absent that I don't know how I would have responded.

What was your most selfish moment?

There were times I felt overloaded by the responsibility and not being able to do more.

Did you feel angry?

No. It was what it was. Anger really had no positive advantage, so for me there was no point in going to anger. There was sadness and emotion, but no anger. Well, except for one time early on in your treatments, the anxiety and frustration was getting to me. So I took Jake to the beach, despite the fact I know dogs are prohibited. Jake was running around and I was trying to enjoy the moment. I saw a man approaching and when he got close he said dogs aren't allowed. I said I would put him on a leash and he said something about protecting some nesting bird. I just exploded. I started screaming at the poor man and continued as I walked away. Every other word was the f bomb. I ranted at him, the county, the world.

Do you have recollections about individual kindnesses?

Mainly, they came from the chemo nurses and the dynamic duo at the front desk. And my friend Steve, who is an oncologist, really reached out. He called every week or so to see how we were both doing. My friend George was also good about calling or emailing.

What else did you find helpful?

One of the principles of Reiki is a prayer you do daily. I reordered it a bit: Just for today do not worry. Just for today try not to grow angry.

How long can you go for without thinking about my cancer?

During the treatment phase it was omnipresent. It was nearly a year before it wasn't a moment-to-moment consideration. It was like a cloud around my head. That didn't clear until the psychic in Honolulu said you do not have cancer anymore. So, that makes it three years.

What was your greatest disappointment?

Telling my parents. I was reaching out to them, but they were in no position to provide the response or support I needed. It was selfish of me to think I would gain solace from them. I shouldn't have told them. All I did was bring pain to them and to me.

Did you find our periodic cry fests to be helpful or cathartic?

No.

So, what does make it better?

A walk on a nice day, talking with you, doing nothing together and doing something for someone else always helps me feel better. Anger or sadness doesn't help. Figuring something out and doing it does.

Do you think we will grow old together?

Yes.

20 AND NOW...

Who knows? The cancer may reemerge. A new cancer could take up residence. The psychics could be right.

What I do know is I have a truly wonderful husband, divine friends and the best dog on the planet. That's plenty.

I don't plan on dying anytime soon, but you never know. Just in case, I'm ending this narrative now. Big tomes are a bit daunting—and horribly time-consuming—especially for us Little C folks living on an often compressed schedule.

ABOUT THE AUTHOR

Phyllis Johnston began her writing career as editor of Mrs. Demby's second grade class newspaper. She dabbled in journalism and public relations before beginning a thirty-year career as a strategic communications consultant, specializing in ballot question campaign management. Luckily, she got the opportunity to spend a year in London and took to writing a daily diary that morphed into her first ebook *Sufferin' London*. An excerpt from the memoir, entitled "Flat Follies," was selected for inclusion in the anthology *A Matter of Choice* published by Seal Press. Her second ebook, *Murder by Choice—A Sister Sleuth Adventure*—was co-written by her Tier One friend Joanne Sandler. A Boston native, Phyllis now lives with her husband Ben and their dog Jake in Sarasota, Florida.